WHAT IS TANTRIC SEX

The Complete Guide to Tantric Sex with Tips for Couples

Table of content

CONCLUSION

Introduction

Tantric sex originates from ancient Hinduism and revolves around sexual practices that focus on creating a deep, intimate connection.

During tantric sex, the aim is to be present in the moment to achieve a sensual and fulfilling sexual experience. Tantric sex encourages people to get to know their own bodies and become in tune with them. By understanding the desire of one's own body, one can incorporate this during sex with a partner. This may lead to greater sexual fulfillment and more intense orgasms. Tantric sex is about honoring one's body and the body of one's partner. By taking time to get to know one's own body as well as that of one's partner, it can help make the experience fulfilling for both people.

When you first start having sex, it can feel a little intimidating. Sure, most people know the missionary style, but where do you go from? We will go through a variety of different sex positions that are great for beginners. This will include places you can try while lying, sitting, standing and kneeling. It should give you an excellent foundation to get started. You can continue to branch from there. It's important to understand that while some positions may be high for you, your partner may not love them. So, trying different things and having an arsenal of different sex positions to work is beneficial for having excellent sex sessions. The massage is incredibly erotic, making sure to soothe the nerves and muscles of the entire body, thus offering the body and mind increased pleasure. You will feel the ancient spiritual arts of sanctifying a deep connection with yourself and with others. With the help of deep, deliberate breathing and visual and mental images, a physical and psychological connection is established. At the same time, you open and stimulate the Chakras, delivering sexual energy and taking you on the path of pure passion.

Many people simply use their imagination to receive intense sexual pleasure. And more and more people are using their creativity and fantasies to spice up their sex life. It is entirely reasonable to fantasize about anything. Choosing your imagination is based on using common sense to determine if it becomes a reality. Sexual fantasy is an excellent way to keep your mind, and perhaps your body motivated whether or not you have sexual fantasies for an entire day, or if you are simply expecting the right individual in the right place and at the right time to act.

Chapter 1:

HOW TANTRIC SEX WORKS AND WHAT IT DOES

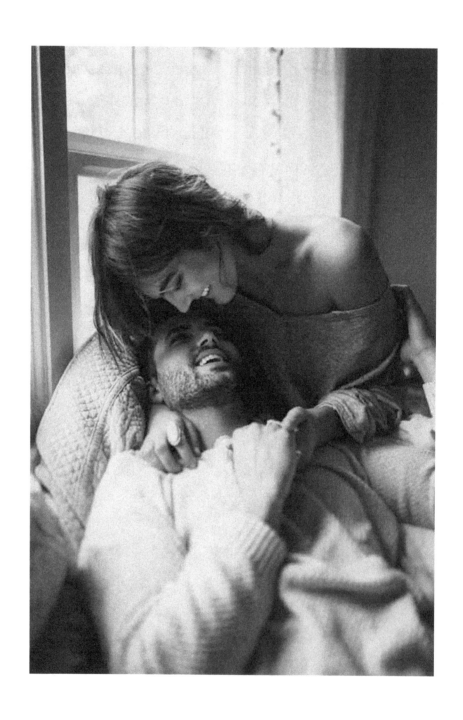

Tantric Sex involves a wide range of erotic activities that not all require the same type of penetration and physical stimulation of the erogenous areas that most individuals associate with Sex.

Tantric Sex often involves the subtle realms with a slow hug, gentle caresses, a presence in the body, and a focus on the energetic movement between the partners' organizations. Sometimes you barely move during tantric Sex, and the emphasis is on the meditative and devotional aspect. You can make love for hours if you relax and take things slow or step up and slow down the action, and the arousal can only keep building.

All sexual energy, however, can be tantric if performed with consciousness. Tantric Sex can immerse you in raw, painful, animal spaces where instinctual body awareness is taking over, and you are blind to pleasure. Domination or obedience can also be tantric.

Some specific acts include tantric massages in which one partner lies down, gets the opportunity for sunlight and sexual energy and sees how he wants to open up through his body. In contrast, the other partner slowly and meditatively moves his hands through his body in so that she can feel every new sensation. People with a penis can pursue practices like edging (near orgasm and back up), which improve their ability to last longer and withhold more pleasure until they reach orgasm.

The respiratory function is also fundamental for tantric Sex; people can use their breath and consciousness to transfer sexual energy through the body, increasing their ability to experience pleasure throughout the body (instead of the joy found exclusively in the genitals).

The purpose of tantric Sex

There can be a variety of sexual goals and expectations, which put some pressure on us and routines and behaviours that keep us stuck in a sexual method. Tantra aims to throw this all out the window and start over with a beginner's mind, to redefine Sex by making it more intimate, binding and playful, rather than a rush to orgasm or a box to check. If you set goals like "eliminate someone" or individually accomplish something, there is infinite room for experimentation and a wide range of what you can do.

And whatever you encounter in orgasms, you can certainly believe there is a lot more to experience with tantric Sex: more intense orgasms, longer-lasting orgasms and full-body orgasms for men, various forms of orgasms, women's orgasms. Multiple, deep conditions of submission, transformative states and states of oneness with your partner and life itself. Several spiritual masters have agreed that orgasm is an experience that gives us a vision of the Lord because, in those times of fellowship, there is a melting of the usual self.

Some other benefits of tantric Sex:

• To get more of what you want in the relationship,

• Liberation of sexual barriers, shame and pain

• To awaken your sexual energy freely to circulate within your body

• To achieve your greatest pleasure and desire

• Whole body and multiple orgasms

• For people with orgasms or who have been interrupted or who suffer from non-ejaculation

• Improved communication

• Longer love sessions, quality of spaciousness and relaxation

• Holistic mind-to-body-to-spirit connection with your partner and yourself

NEOTANTRA AND CLASSIC TANTRA

Tantra comes from Hindu, Buddhist and Jain styles and texts from at least the seventh century, if not earlier. However, usually, when people from Western Europe use the term "tantra", they are talking about the area of "neotantra". There are several nuanced and rigorous religious paths of "modern tantra" aimed at complete awakening and spiritual enlightenment. Among these are Kashmir Shaivism, a branch of Kashmir and the spiritual traditions of India, and the Vajrayana Buddhist path from India and Tibet. Both approaches also require serious study and personal devotion, reflection, and can include numerous ceremonial elements, such as the use of mantras, visualizations, and worship of divinity. Sexual energy was a minor part of the exercise and was only open to advanced students.

neotantra, however, has evolved over the past 150 years and primarily aims to strengthen intimacy and attachment, deeper bonds with one's body and feelings, healing pain and barriers, and opening up greater orgasmic bliss. Some fundamental principles of classical Tantra have profoundly influenced this collection of teachings. Still, it is essential to recognize that many of what is learned and practised by contemporary tantric sexual practitioners are "old practices".

Let's talk about the Capgras illusion.

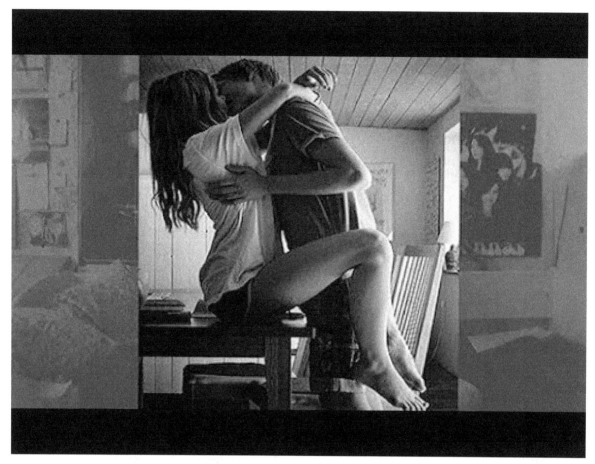

Now, you are probably wondering what it is. For you to truly understand the concept, we need to delve into the complex world of the mind. The Capgras delusion is a psychological condition in which the sufferer believes that impostors have replaced his friends, relatives, spouse or other people close to him (including pets). No matter how hard you try to convince them of their delusion, they cannot easily let go of this belief. It sticks deeply into their mind. People suffer from delusion not only due to psychological conditions - brain dysfunction and injury can also cause these symptoms.

Imagine thinking that the people close to you are not real. It's like watching those horror movies where otherworldly beings have replaced all people. The only difference is that in the case of the Capgras illusion, everything exists only in the person's head. People are real. Relationships are real. But the person suffering from the Capgras delusion cannot believe it.

For example, this person might have a conversation with their parents, where mom and dad use family photos and other cues to try to explain to the sufferer that they are related. But no explanation or proof can erase the illusion. The belief has penetrated deep into the sufferer's mind, and he refuses to let go.

Why did we raise the Capgras illusion? We want to discuss its cause. No, we are not talking about psychological or physical damage; instead, we are looking at the consequences these problems can bring.

You see, people suffering from the Capgras delusion have a damaged emotional centre. This means that the emotional response we feel when we look at our friends, family members, and people close to us does not exist with Capgras delusion sufferers.

We often underestimate our emotional responses. We think they are simply by-products of what we think of the other person. But our emotions are powerful. And they are a vital part of how we make connections. Just like the way the Capgras delusion empties the feelings behind the relationships we feel with others, dull and uninteresting sex is what happens when our emotional responses to him are inhibited or, in some cases, interrupted.

Sex is not just a physical act. It is an exciting journey. You and your partner may seek more intimacy in your relationship. You may be reflecting on how best to develop deeper and more meaningful communications, or perhaps even trying to transfer sincere feelings to each other during sex. As you reach a deeper level of connection with your partner, you come to a point where your relationship becomes more profound.

Tantra is the key to opening the doors of intimacy, emotions and even the spiritual journey. But each key has an origin. After all, it has to be forged somewhere and with a purpose.

Let's dive into the origin of Tantra.

Chapter 2

HOW DOES TANTRIC SEX VARY FROM REGULAR SEX?

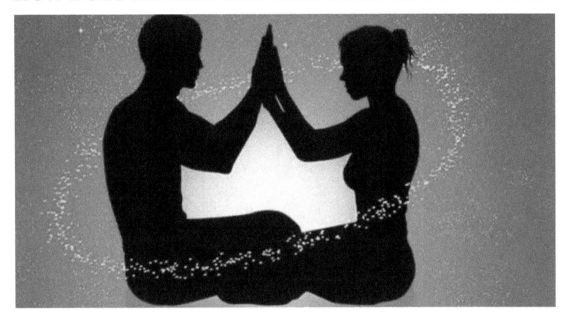

You've heard of tantric sex. Unfortunately, however, this is generally encased in a mysterious cloud that gives many people more thrills than a good understanding. It often feels like a topic is being moved into a sacred / forbidden position that no one wants to come forward; sit on the surface of something so fascinating and productive?

It does not mean that it is dirty just because it contains the word sex, and the word tantric means neither mystical nor strange. We expose the main difference between this ancient sexual form and what most people do. Before that, though, it's nice to shed some light on some key aspects.

The word Tantra has different roots in different traditional Indian languages, but most sources agree that it usually means extension, expansion or release. Tantric sex has been a part of Indian Ayurvedic culture for some 1,500 years, as have meditation and yoga. The numerous erotic sculptures in the temples show their importance to Indian culture. See gender as another form of spirituality.

Although regular sex usually goes through three stages: foreplay, intercourse, and completion, tantric sex does not advance linearly. It is not orgasm oriented! Tantric prostitutes tend not to see orgasm as the primary source of pleasure.

How do they do it?

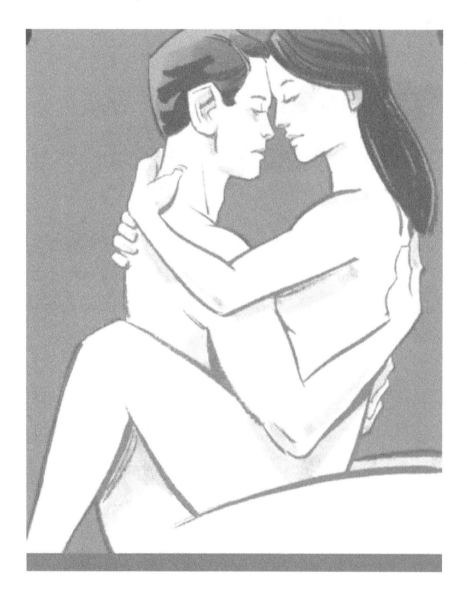

In tantric sex, the couple tries to connect with their sexual energy more intensely than just the physical level. We try to psychologically extend this power from the genitals to the whole body so that every point can be a source of fun. We synchronize our breathing and focus on combining with the power of partners for a deeper connection. In this method, maintaining eye contact is critical.

A tantric sex session can last for several hours because physical energy or orgasm does not culminate. Instead, the couple is immersed in a state of imagination, which can cycle in any direction except on a long finish. You may be in a relationship or just touching yourself with the same intensity of pleasure. Tantric sex couples experience waves of orgasms.

Tantric sex seeks the highest and purest relationship through heat. This sounds like tantric sex, healthy sex; yoga is the standard practice of gymnastics. The mind, spirit and power are involved as much as the body.

Wasn't sex supposed to be a vessel of what we call love? Why is love not the highest manifestation of the spirit? The tantric genre is based on these very fundamental concepts.

Chapter 3

BENEFITS OF TANTRIC SEX

You can improve your sexual health naturally through tantric yoga and gender. Tantric yoga offers many exercises that lead to a stable and blissful life, including a powerful combination of asanas, mantras, mudras, bandhas and chakras. Tantric sex is a slow type of intimacy that can enhance closeness and a connection between the mind and body, which often results in intense orgasms. This combination, with a secure connection between body, mind and spirit along with frequent and intense sexual orgasms, should allow loving couples to increase pineal and hypo-physical secretion.

- Tantric sex improves sexual health

Many say that Tantric sex has a rejuvenating effect, improving the sexual health of both men and women. Frequent orgasms can alter body chemistry, like one of the brain wave simulations. Depression and stress can go away. A woman's sexual health can be significantly improved.

The tantric gender can be affected by the endocrine glands for more HGH, dopamine, DHEA and testosterone. Brain chemistry can be changed. Scientific and medical studies have shown that gender significantly improves health by improving blood circulation, detoxifying the body's breathing, and improving cardiovascular, endocrine/immune and nerve functions. For example, a study conducted by Wilkes University found that making love produces an antibody called immunoglobulin A or IgA at least twice a week that can protect the body from disease.

- Orgasms that strengthen the immune system

Orgasms can minimize anxiety and make you feel happier and happier. Others claim it can also extend your life, boost your immune system, and improve your overall health. To confirm these findings, however, further clinical studies are needed. Can sexual exposure to sperm fight depression and raise the mood in both women and men? It may also be found that risky and unsafe sex can lead to depression. In contrast, safe sex can provide spirit, emotional connections, and intimacy, according to a report by Rebecca Burch. Therefore, men and women can significantly benefit from increasing sexual quantity and quality in a discreet, healthy and natural way through tantric sex.

Possible benefits of constant orgasms, women's health, and tantric sex

Frequent orgasms can benefit a woman's sexual health. There is this vast difference between a normal orgasm and a tantric orgasm. Frequent orgasms last for a short time and remain isolated in the sexual organs. Theoretically, tantric sexual orgasms involve the whole body, mind and spirit and last for hours.

According to ancient traditions, to obtain the benefits of a tantric orgasm, shakti or power, and kundalini, each of the chakras must penetrate the ascending spinal cord (energy vortexes in the subtle body). It must enter the central nervous system of the brain and the endocrine site: the hypothalamus and pituitary that regulate changes in our sexual health.

Tantric sex devotees claim that strong and robust orgasms increase the level of the orgasm hormone, oxytocin. We also agree that oxytocin levels and your orgasms affect your mood, your enthusiasm, your social skills and your emotions.

Chapter 4

It's not just about sex.

Tantra was founded in Hinduism and Buddhism, but it is not a religion by nature. To understand this better, let's take an example. Suppose a non-religious couple finds some of the Bible's inspired values and teachings. They decide that those values are positive influences and create a set of guidelines based on them, which are then used in their lives to improve their way of life.

Here is the question: Are the guidelines established by the couple a "religion", since they are based on the Bible? If this couple decides to support the needy in their area because they have read a section of the Bible on alms to the poor, does it automatically mean that their guidelines are a religion in their own right? Sure, we can all agree that they have religious influences, but they are not a religion of their own.

Tantra follows a similar guideline, where it takes all the positive influences of Hinduism and Buddhism to create a vibrant and colourful tradition. As we explained earlier, Hinduism uses a caste system, while Tantra abolishes any system that segregates people into groups. Suppose the best way to say this is that Tantra doesn't copy directly from Hinduism or Buddhism - it takes the best lessons from the two religions. It incorporates them into its foundations in a meaningful way.

The word "Tantra" means "loom" in Sanskrit. There are numerous explanations to define the meaning of the word fully; however, the most common theory is that it should be a play on words.

To understand the pun, one should return to the sutras. As mentioned earlier, the sutras are ancient texts. The word sutra translates to "thread," referring to a single thread of thought that creates the texts in Hinduism, Buddhism and Jainism.

Therefore, if the sutra is regarded as a single thread, Tantra is the loom that produces these threads, ultimately leading to a collection of thoughts.

The idea behind the pun was that if religions created threads of thought, then they had a rather narrow view of theory. Tantra, on the other hand, has taken all the strings to build a frame, broadening the horizons of thought and allowing people to see the bigger picture.

So what kind of thoughts did Tantra spread?

Regardless of where you practise Tantra or who you teach, the commonalities shared by the various forms remain the same. They include the following:

• An embodiment of the act of awareness. People learned to bring their thoughts into the present, where they could calmly recognize the thoughts, feelings and physical sensations that flowed through their being.

• The act of deepening one's awareness to understand oneself more clearly. This allows people better to diagnose mental, emotional and even physical problems.

• A rejection of arbitrary rules established by religions and cultures. Tantra often encouraged people to wonder if they were pleased with the way things are. Do they feel comfortable with specific rules that they are encouraged to follow simply because they are part of a particular culture or religion?

• Acceptance of people, regardless of their background. This means that Tantra saw all people as one, irrespective of their race, sex, nationality or other character traits.

• Unlimited and unmediated access to the divine. This means that you are not allowed access to divinity or the Almighty simply because you follow a particular religion. If you are looking for divine influence in your life, then you are free to seek it in Tantra.

• A belief that sensual and bodily experiences are nothing to be ashamed of or reject; instead, they are part of the package to help us achieve peace and spirituality.

Tantric teachings have been prevalent in the exploration of sex. But tradition is not just a sexual guide, unlike the works of the Kama Sutra. Indeed, there is still a growing debate as to whether sex was also the main focus of Tantra. Some believe it has had increasing importance in the tradition, while others support it. However, there is no doubt that the main focus of Tantra has never been sex, but an individual's spiritual journey.

So why do many people often relate Tantra to sexuality, even though the tradition contains numerous essential teachings? Although there are many reasons for this question, a prevailing theory is the broad and open view of sexuality in Tantra. He doesn't disapprove of sex or rejects conversations about it. It accepts sexuality as part of the human experience and even elevates it to a spiritual state.

It's about the individual.

Tantra means making many changes in people's lives. It is about being individual and improving their spiritual, emotional and mental states.

• Awaken the spirituality of individuals. It allows people to truly open their minds and examine their lives in new and profound ways.

• It allows people to explore sex in ways they never thought possible. This strengthens relationships not only on a physical level but on an emotional and spiritual level.

• Let's not forget the fact that tantric life can also relieve stress. When you are present at the spiritual level prescribed by Tantra, you are calmer in real life. You have more control over your emotions and stay focused when engaged inactivity.

● Tantra also promotes your general well-being. You feel like a new person as if you are being held captive inside a shell that has now opened, giving you the power to glimpse the world with freedom and clarity.

● Thanks to tantra practices, you can also unplug from your daily routine. It allows you to relax pleasantly. Who says you can't relax and have fun at the same time? Tantra allows people to live their lives with more excitement, peace, joy and fulfilment. That said, let's venture into a vibrant and sensual tradition.

Now we will understand more about Tantra its

Chapter 5

Main areas of interest

Now that you are familiar with the concept of Tantra, you will probably want to learn more about tantric sex. However, you must start at the fundamental level to enter the world of Tantra. Let's start with the basics, looking at specific concepts you should be aware of and suggesting exercises that you might find useful on your Tantric journey.

Opposites attract

We have already examined the yin and yang aspects of Tantra. But how does this manifest itself in Tantra itself? One of the most famous images of yin and yang is manifested in Hindu mythology in the form of the god Shiva and the goddess Shakti. These two entities are considered to be the source of the energies of the universe. For this reason, the union of these two influential figures from Hindu mythology is responsible for manifesting the desire that exists between you and your partner. It allows you to put yourself as god and goddess of your own lives. Just like how yin can become yang and vice versa, Shiva completes the powers of Shakti - and the other way around. You may find this divine couple depicted in numerous positions, as they hug, dance, or are simply physically close to each other. In some depictions, you may also find Shakti wrapping her legs around Shiva's hips. The pure sexual energy between them is meant to show their love and admiration for each other. However, the most popular position of the two deities is their dancing form, which is considered the most sacred. This not only indicates that the two gods are able to release their energies, but they can also achieve harmony with each other and enlightenment in their lives.

But what does all this have to do with Tantra?

A lot. Using Shiva and Shakti as inspiration, couples are encouraged to understand each other. This is because Shiva and Shakti are not the perfect couples, despite being powerful deities. But the secret of their love and happiness is based on the fact that they try to understand each other without restrictions or barriers.

Figure 7: Shiva and Shakti are often depicted embraced and, at times, locked in an erotic pose.

You and your partner must be the Shakti and Shiva in your relationship. As we learned earlier, yin and yang are two forms on the same plane. But merely believing in yin and yang doesn't automatically clear the barriers in your relationship.

Your first step is to start communicating with each other about the divisions plaguing your relationship. You two have opposite energies. After all, when one is yin, the other is yang. This does not mean that one is good while the other is bad. It merely suggests that during your relationship, you both automatically alternated between yin and yang. However, you may not have done it together. It's like dancing with each other while keeping a distance of one and a half meters between you. You could still say that you are both dancing, but you have no physical contact, thus removing the grace, power and impact that a real dance should have. Look at the traits you two have. You may find that some of them are somewhat stereotyped, while others may surprise you. Once you discover these traits, you should focus on hugging them and loving each other despite their presence. If you or your partner find that you have specific characteristics that might be causing the other person discomfort, try to understand and work with these traits. When you realize that the differences you two possess could be the attraction that draws you together, then you may learn to accept each other with all your heart truly.

Bring little signs of love back into your relationship. It could be something as simple as giving yourself a loving nickname or making small gestures and gestures to show your appreciation for each other. Don't plan these gestures. Run them whenever you can. Surprise each other.

Practice Tantra

Various practices will help you initiate tantric sex. These exercises will enhance the ecstasy you achieve during your sexual experiences. At the same time, they allow you to remove any mental blocks, such as stress. We recommend that you take the time to practice and master these techniques to get the most out of tantric sex. Don't worry - these are techniques that won't take long to master, as you'll soon find out.

Your first exercise is learning the art of breathing correctly.

The breath of life

When you breathe properly, you are supplying your body with the necessary amount of oxygen it needs. But that's not all you are doing. As your body receives oxygen, it also circulates sensuality and emotions. How is this achieved? When the body receives adequate oxygen, all of its parts begin to function in harmony. This makes you more active, even during sex. At the same time, the brain becomes better able to handle your emotions correctly. If you start paying attention to your breathing, you may simply notice that you are holding your breath too much. You have to relax this tension in your body, and the only way to do this is through breathing.

Tantric breathing

Take about 15 minutes to breathe deeply and gently. To do this correctly, use the following steps:

- **Step 1:** Sit comfortably in a cross-legged position. If you find it uncomfortable to cross your legs, use a chair.
- **Step 2:** Now take a deep breath. As you inhale, count to six. As you inhale, imagine your breath reaching down to the lower genitals.
- **Step 3:** Hold your breath for four seconds.
- **Step 4:** Finally, release your breath as you count to seven.

During the breathing exercise, clear your mind to experience sexual thoughts about your partner. However, don't dwell on them. As soon as you notice an idea, let it fade away. Don't ignore them, instead acknowledge them, thinking about the excitement they bring you and then move on to the next thought.

The well of breath

This exercise is designed to improve your lung capacity, allowing you to breathe deeply during sex. The primary technique is to fill the lungs with as much oxygen as possible. At the same time, exercise will allow you to manage the sounds you make while having sex.

To perform this exercise, get in a comfortable position. Ideally, we recommend sitting in a chair as it allows you to keep your arms in a warm place. But if you feel like sitting on the floor, contact-free to do so. For this exercise, you need to keep your arms at your side (that's why we recommend a chair).

When you are ready, follow these steps:

- **Step 1:** Get as much air into your lungs as possible. Imagine your lungs as a balloon that inflates that can expand significantly. When you inhale, make as much noise as possible with your breath. Your inhalation should be audible.

- **Step 2:** When you feel you have reached the limits of the capacity of your lungs, hold your breath for a few seconds.
- **Step 3:** When you release your breath, exhale with some force. It should sound like a Boeing 747 about to launch into the sky, or at least like a gust of wind is escaping your lungs.

Another crucial benefit of this exercise is that it lowers the stress levels in your body. This is important because you shouldn't be in a negative mental state during tantric sex. Training also allows you to employ breathing techniques during sex, allowing you to take your mind away from orgasm thoughts to focus on the experience itself, allowing you to delay orgasm as much as possible to enjoy a prolonged sexual experience.

Chapter 6

Yoga-ta Do It!

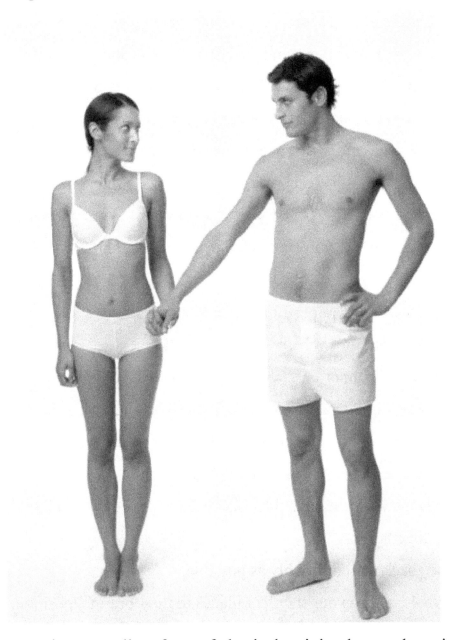

Yoga is an excellent form of physical activity that works to improve your
emotional, physical and mental states. The yoga poses you will learn in this section
will help you improve your stamina and overall health. When you combine these
poses with breathing exercises, you will have a powerful tool for enhancing your
sex life.

We recommend that you and your partner practice yoga together. This way, you can help each other improve poses. Plus, practising together allows you to increase the levels of comfort and intimacy you share. As you start helping each other out, you become less afraid to reveal your flaws and discomforts. You and your partner become encouraged to communicate problems. That way, if any of you have any questions during sex, they won't hesitate to talk about it. Remember that you don't always have to be perfect. Tantra means discovering each other. The beginnings will be awkward and probably full of missteps. But try to enjoy those moments! Feel free to laugh at your mistakes. They allow you to connect with your partner on such a deep level that you feel like you are talking to your other half.

Head Lift

To perform this pose, start in a standing position. Keep your posture relaxed, making sure your back doesn't lean forward.

- **Step 1:** Tilt your head up, but not face up ultimately. You should look up diagonally. Stretch your neck slightly, as if someone is gently lifting your head. Don't stretch so far that you end up feeling uncomfortable. Make sure you keep your mouth closed to make sure you are breathing through your nose only.

- **Step 2:** As you inhale, move your shoulder blades back. It should feel like you're trying to put them together.

Push your shoulder blades back as comfortably as possible.

- **Step 3:** As you exhale, return your shoulder blades to their original position.

- **Step 4:** Make sure your feet aren't moving and are planted firmly on the floor.

Upward dog

For this pose, you should ideally lie face down. You can choose to lie on the floor, on a mat or the bed. We recommend one of the first two options to avoid any back strain.

- **Step 1:** Extend your body, allowing your stomach to touch the floor.

- **Step 2:** Bring your arms close to your shoulders, so it looks like you're about to do push-ups.

- **Step 3:** Take a deep breath and, as you inhale, lift your upper body off the ground and look forward. At this point, your back should be curved, with the legs as straight as they can be.

- **Step 4:**Maintain the pose for as long as possible. As you get better, you will be able to keep it longer. Ideally, you should aim for at least 60 seconds, but don't worry if you find that you need to stop after less than

10 seconds. The idea is not to punish yourself or become a yoga master.

Cat pose

From dogs to cats: the transition from dog-up to cat pose is smooth. When you have completed the Upward Dog Pose, gently relax into a face-down position. Take a moment to catch your breath if you want. Again, don't try too hard. Take it easy as you move from one pose to another. To move into the cat position, start in a relaxed position after completing the upward dog.

- **Step 1:** Position yourself on your hands and knees in what is commonly referred to as the "table" position. Your hands should be pressed firmly to the floor, and your knees should be directly under your hips. Don't turn your head; look straight at the level.

- **Step 2:**Inhale. As you take air into your lungs, bend your back towards the ceiling (or towards the sky, if you are practising yoga outdoors). You should bring your head a little closer to the floor, but don't tuck your chin towards your chest. At this point, you will still be looking at the storey, but at a slight angle. You may also have a view of your knees. If you can't see them, don't push it.

- **Step 3:** Hold your breath for a few seconds and then release. As you exhale, return to your original position. Remember not to hold your breath for too long, a couple of seconds at the most. Don't even force yourself to stay in the hunched position for too long. Do the exercise at least 20 times.

Position of the corpse

This yoga posture has a sombre but appropriate name. Also called savasana, this pose mimics a resting corpse. The idea behind the pose is to stay as still as possible. Once the cat pose is complete, lie on your back.

- **Step 1:** Let the arms and legs fall naturally - the arms should be at the sides, and the legs positioned hip-width apart. This pose is meant to relax you as much as possible, so stay comfortable.

- **Step 2:** The palms of the hands and toes should be facing the ceiling or sky. When you're comfortable enough, start breathing normally, don't take deep breaths. Simply relax, allowing yourself to melt into the floor or ground beneath you.

- **Step 3:** Now, take three deep breaths before returning your breathing to normal. Lie in this position for about five minutes. Don't worry if you hear thoughts going through your mind. Focus on your breathing. You may get distracted, but don't feel impatient. Regardless of how many distractions you face, calmly recognize it and resume breathing.

When you have completed the Corpse Pose, you can return your body to its original position. Take three deep breaths and finish the yoga pose (or session, if you've done all of the poses mentioned in this section).

We recommend that you practice all the yoga poses mentioned here. Don't worry if you can't perfect the poses on the first try or keep them for long. As soon as you feel uncomfortable in one particular posture, move on to the next. Take a short break between them if it helps.

Chapter 7

Tantric exercises

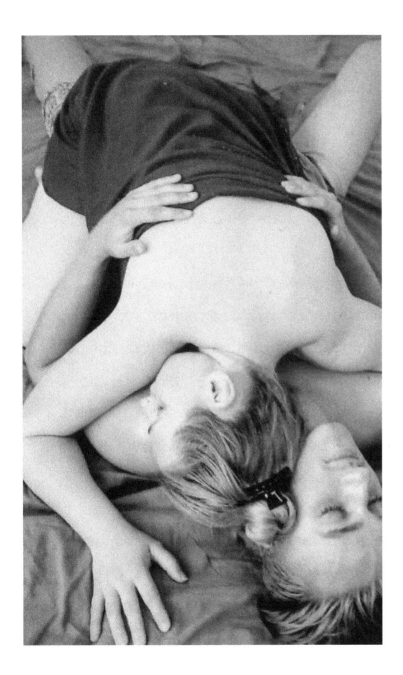

You can make your sexual experiences even better by improving your physical state, and the best way to do this is by exercising. If you already have an exercise regimen in place, you don't need to interrupt your current routine. Think of the following tips as bonuses that can improve your physical well-being.

However, if you are not currently following any exercise routines, consider incorporating them into your life, ideally by doing them daily.

Shoulder support

This exercise is especially useful for men and women to easily assume some of the tantric poses mentioned later in this book. At the same time, it improves the flexibility of your body.

- **Step 1:** Lie on the floor or a mat. Make sure your legs are straight and your arms with palms facing down at your side.

- **Step 2:** Slowly raise your leg, bringing it to a 90-degree angle. Make sure your upper torso is still on the floor.

- **Step 3:** Now lift your legs a little higher so that your lower back is also raised. Place your hands on your back so you can support yourself and hold the position for as long as possible - ideally, for 60 seconds, but don't feel compelled to keep the job if you feel uncomfortable.

If you are unable to perform this exercise comfortably, do not strain your back as you try it. Go through the steps slowly. You can check if you are ready to complete the task by first trying to perform the steps slowly until you can maintain a comfortable position. For example, you might start by lifting your legs until they are positioned at a 45-degree angle. If you can handle the situation comfortably, bring your legs closer to the 90-degree corner.

Practice doing the exercise until you can hold the final position for at least 30 seconds. Don't be discouraged if it takes you more than a month to complete the move. After all, you are not competing for a prize; you are merely improving flexibility for Tantra. Practising the exercise every day helps you become more flexible, so don't feel like you're not making progress.

Laying the boat

This is a slightly more straightforward exercise than the previous one. However, the challenge lies in maintaining the final position.

- **Step 1:** Lie on your back on the floor or mat with your legs extended and your hands at your sides.
- **Step 2:** Slowly raise your legs to a 45-degree angle. Keep them in that position.
- **Step 3:** Raise your hands so that your fingers point towards your feet. All you need to do now is to hold this pose for as long as possible. Keep practising until you can last three minutes.

Exercise for three-legged dogs

The main benefit of this exercise is to strengthen and improve the hamstrings. Not only will this benefit your tantric sexual experience, but it will also help you in your daily life.

- **Step 1:** To start, lie on your stomach on the floor or a mat. Keep your hands positioned at your sides, as if you are going to do a push-up. Curl your toes inward so that your lower body is balanced on the base of your toes. When you bend your toes, you avoid balancing on your toes, which could cause injury or an accident.
- **Step 2:** Lift your glutes towards the ceiling. You should reach a position where your body forms a triangle with the floor or ground as its base. Push yourself up using your hands and feet.
- **Step 3:** Now lift your leg straight up, bringing your knee closer to your chest. Lift your leg as high as you can, don't force it. Once the pin has reached its maximum angle, return it to its original position.
- **Step 4:** Perform the previous move with the other leg, making sure you don't push yourself to lift the leg too close to your body if you are unable to do so.
- **Step 5:** Try to do 20 reps on each leg if possible.

table

This is such an underrated (and quite challenging to perform) exercise that it helps you strengthen your core. To complete the task correctly, use the following steps.

- **Step 1:** Lie face down and assume a push-up position. Make sure you are comfortable before moving on to the next step.

- **Step 2:** Place your forearms on the floor and lift yourself, balancing your lower body on your toes. To relieve discomfort, be sure to bend your toes inward and put pressure on the base of your toes.

- **Step 3:** Make sure your elbows are as close to a 90-degree angle as possible. Maintain the position for as long as possible, aiming for at least two minutes.

Jumping Jacks

It is essential that the blood pump throughout the body. To do this, and to burn calories along the way, you should consider jumping jacks. When it comes to Tantra, jumping studs improve your stamina.

You may already be familiar with this exercise, but following these steps will ensure that you are doing them correctly.

- **Step 1:** Start from a standing position, standing with your legs together and your hands by your side.

- **Step 2:** When ready, bend your knees slightly to give yourself a push. Jump into the air, but not too high.

- **Step 3:** As you jump, spread your legs, so they're shoulder-width apart. At the same time, bring your arms above your head. Some people think that your arms should be straight when they are above your head, but this is not required.

- **Step 4:** Return to your original position and immediately go to the next repetition of the jumping jack. Continue until you perform 50 repetitions of the exercise.

Don't worry if you can't hit 50 reps. Focus on doing the jumping jack correctly.

lunges

Lunges are simple exercises that work effectively on the hamstrings, glutes, and hips. Improve flexibility in the lower body while strengthening your legs. They are also an ideal exercise to improve your stamina.

Here's how to make the lunges:

- **Step 1:** Stand with your feet slightly apart. For best results, align your feet with your hips. Relax your body, and make sure your spine is straight.

- **Step 2:** Step forward with one leg. Transfer your weight forward so that when you take the stage, your heel touches the floor first.

- **Step 3**: Lower your body until your thigh is parallel to the floor. Your shin area should be vertical or as close as possible - as long as your knee is past the toe, you are good to go.

- **Step 4:** Return to the original position, then move to the next leg and repeat the procedure. Do 20 reps on each leg, but relax if you can't reach your goal.

If you think your mobility is slowing, you can tap the floor lightly with the knee of the other leg. For example, if you are doing the above exercise on your right leg, you will find yourself balanced on the toes of your left leg. You may notice that the knee of the left leg will be close to the floor. Bring your knee to the ground and give it a light nudge before standing up to your original position.

With the exercises above, you can improve your core, get blood pumping throughout your body, increase endurance, and improve your flexibility. If you wish, you can also do some jumping jacks before having sex to get the blood flowing throughout your body. Rather than doing 50 reps, stick to 10. You just need to energize your body, don't get tired before having sex!

Chapter 8

orgasm

Now that we understand intimacy and the different types of privacy that can exist in relationships, we'll see how you can rekindle your desire for fire in your relationship and with your partner. One of the best ways for a very familiar couple to revive their sex life is to rediscover sex from the beginning, again, with their partner. While you may have a lot of experience when it comes to having sex, there may still be some things that each of you doesn't know. This could be in terms of the other person's body, in terms of the G-spots of both females and males, or how everything works from an anatomical point of view. Before moving on to other ways to rekindle your sexual fire,

Female sexual anatomy

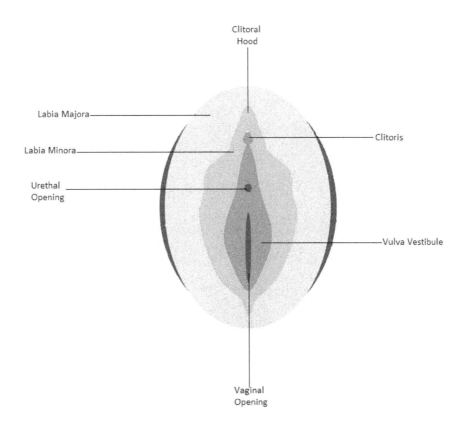

To lead a woman to orgasm, you will need to know the female body and all the places that, when stimulated, will make a woman feel pleasure. Whether you are a woman or a male with a female partner, both genders can benefit from learning more about the female body. The two main points that we will look at are the clitoris and the G-spot. These two places both have great potential in terms of bringing a woman to be intense and mind-blowing orgasms.

The clitoris

The clitoris is the place that many people know as the point of stimulation, which is the easiest way to give a woman an orgasm. The clitoris is located very close to the vagina. It's a small, bean-like structure that has many, many nerve endings, which is why it can easily lead to female pleasure. To find it, start by placing a hand on the pelvic area, with your fingers towards the vagina. A woman can do it alone, or a man can do it to find the woman's clitoris. Slowly move your hand down, using your fingers to feel around. As you wrap your fingers under her, between her legs, look for a small, lump-like structure. It's in a slightly different spot, covered in varying amounts of layers and different sizes on each woman, so explore between her legs to find it. It will be towards the front of her body, right where her vaginal lips begin. On some women, you may even be able to see it with your eyes if there aren't as many layers of labia covering it.

The clitoris is said to be the female penis. This is because it gets bigger and swollen when a woman is horny. It will be easier to find her clit if she is on. The clitoris is much larger than it looks, and this is because it extends inside the woman's body. Only a small part is on the outside of the body, but its size is the reason why there are so many nerve endings located inside and why stimulating it will lead to such intense pleasure.

Once you find your clitoris, you can then stimulate it to give yourself or your woman an orgasm. Start by gently placing two fingers on it and applying gentle pressure. Rub by moving your fingers in small circles, making sure you are kind. Keep doing this, and she should start getting more excited the more you do it. By rubbing the clitoris, you will be able to stimulate the whole clitoris, even the part that you cannot see, and this will cause the woman to start getting wet in her vagina.

The point G.

The G-spot is a lesser-known spot on the clitoris, but a woman can experience an extreme amount of pleasure if this spot is stimulated. To find this spot, you'll need to insert a finger into her vagina. It is best to try to find this spot after stimulating the clitoris a little because then her vagina will have started to get wet as it lubricates itself to prepare for penetration. You can use this to your advantage as it will make penetration more enjoyable for her and reduce the friction of the entire vaginal area in general. When the vagina gets very wet, it can lubricate the whole vaginal area, including the clitoris, which will make it easier to stimulate the clitoris as well. No friction means smooth sliding, which results in pleasure and pain-free. When it's wet enough, slide a finger inside her vagina while she is lying on her back a woman can also do it alone and make a "come here" motion with her finger to move it towards her navel. Feel around in this area, and when you feel an uneven or rough surface, this is the G-spot. Just like the clitoris, the G-spot is slightly different for each woman, but they can all be in the same general area. The G-spot will have different sizes for different women, so keep this in mind when trying to find it. But they can all be in the same general area. The G-spot will have different sizes for different women, so keep this in mind when trying to find it. But they can all be in the same general area. G-spot will have different size for different women,

The reason the G-spot can give a woman intense pleasure is that it is connected to the clitoris. Inside the body, where the clitoris extends into the woman, it meets the vagina, and this is where the GSpot is located. This thin wall between them allows pressure and stimulation to travel between them, so you're essentially stimulating your clitoris as well when you're enjoying her G-spot.

To please a woman by stimulating her G-spot, you will have to press it over and over until orgasm is achieved. This can be done using the fingers, penis or sex toys of various types. For now, we will look at the fingers and the penis. Stimulating this point with your fingers is quite simple as you will have a lot of control and will be able to feel around to see if you are in the right spot. When you've found the G-spot with your fingers, press it gently with your fingertips and avoid curling your fingers too much because you don't want your nails to scratch the inside of her vagina. Press your fingertips on her G-spot with light pressure, but enough for her to feel what you are doing. Keep doing this, and you should contact her vagina getting wetter and wetter. While you do it, you can increase the stimulation speed if you wish. Communicate with her to see what she wants you to do faster, slower, harder, lighter, deeper, more superficial. A woman can do the same to herself in the bedroom.

Similarly, I run a finger inside your vagina with some lube or after getting wet a little while watching porn or massaging your clit. Then, move your finger to the front of the body and look for the spot. Once found, continue to stimulate it by putting pressure on it over and over again. It should feel good and get better and better as you do it. Eventually, the pleasure will increase until you feel like you are about to orgasm.

The penis can also stimulate the G-spot, but it's a bit more difficult as there won't be as much control as there is when using your fingers. Try to choose a position that will have the curve of the penis aligned with the front of the vaginal wall, and this will give you the best chance of hitting the G-spot. For now, though, know where the G-spot is and how to get pleasure from a woman at that point is a great start to be able to give her a fantastic orgasm.

Chapter 9

Male sexual anatomy

The penis

As we know, the male sexual organ is the penis. A man can reach orgasm by having his penis massaged, sucked, kissed, or stimulated in many other ways. While you can't quickly tell when a woman is aroused, it's easy to tell when a man is aroused because his penis will get erect. This happens because then he can have sex with it - think about how difficult it would be to have penetrative sex with a soft penis. When a man watches porn, sees a beautiful woman, or is touched in the right way, he will become erect. Then, by repeatedly sliding his penis into a vagina, in a sex toy like a Fleshlight or by having it stroked with his hand, he can finally reach orgasm. Every man's penis has a different shape and a different size,

The testicles

A man's testicles may appear to be there only to supply sperm for ejaculation, but they are also susceptible to erogenous zones for a man. If a man's testicles are stimulated, this can make him very aroused and can make him erect if he wasn't already. A man's testicles can be stimulated during oral sex, during manual labour, or during sex in certain positions, and this will only add to the pleasure he is already experiencing having his penis stimulated in some way.

If you've ever had your testicles bumped the wrong way, it caused you a lot of pain for those few minutes later. Think about that level of pain but in terms of pleasure instead. This is what we want to unlock for you in your testicles—this level of sensation, but conversely, intense pleasure instead of severe pain. Gently stroking your testicles with warm hands will get them used to touch each other, so they don't cling and hug your body too tightly. Gently rubbing the scrotum and massaging the testicles will add to any sexual activity already in progress. They can also be stimulated with the mouth during oral sex. The woman can move to her testicles and gently suck or lick them to give a different sensation, that of warm moisture on sensitive skin.

A man can stimulate his testicles while masturbating for added pleasure. If you are a man and have never tried it, add it to your next masturbation session. Using one hand to stroke your penis and the other to massage your testicles will add a new dimension to your self-love sessions. Try it in the shower with a partner or without to enjoy the warmth or water mixed with a massage and stimulation of the penis. You'll never go back.

Pre-sexual rituals

Most couples who have lived together for a long time love each other but tend to stop making love. Some couples continue to love each other despite the absence of sex. They say marriage does not suffer from a lack of sex. How do they hold the flame when the desire is gone?

Some couples don't even remember the last time they made love. There is a story of a couple in my neighbourhood, Mathew and Eva, around 48, married for 21 years, happy parents of two children. By their admission, they gradually put their sexuality aside. This does not prevent them from laughing together, from taking to the streets or from sleeping against each other.

Without claiming him or being part of the "no sex" movement in recent years, Mathew and Eva have found a marital balance that belongs to them, refusing to make this lack of jokes a "problem". A less rare choice than it seems, the heart has its reasons which the body sometimes ignores. Now some might ask, to love without making love, is it possible? How does sexual desire arise? What is the physical attraction of men and women?

Often it is after childbirth, the loss of a loved one or a job, bereaved situations that numb the libidinal sexual drive and, in the event of unemployment, damage self-esteem that the couple stops all sexual activity. Hugs become scarce until they disappear entirely from the marital landscape. Because the less we make love, the less desire there is, as the sex drive is self-powered, more like a battery. Our partner stimulates our appetite not only because he is beautiful or beautiful, feels good and is intelligent, but because he occupies a special place in our psychic organization.

According to Freudian theory, unconsciously, a woman often sees in her partner the man who will make her become a mother or a saviour who has symbolically killed her innocence to free her from being a child. A man tends to see in his partner, which will allow him to surpass his father. Therefore, spouses have to invent another sexuality. So the issues of motherhood and paternity disappeared. This is also the case with menopause. They have to reconstruct the inner scenarios, this time focusing mainly on just having fun and the challenging psychic task if their relationship with pleasure is tinged with guilt.

According to most couples, physical distance doesn't happen overnight. Most women always say that it is after their last birth that the rhythm of making love starts to get boring. "Not only was I unable to enjoy myself, but I was in pain. Mathew ended up afraid of making me suffer, Eva said. So he stopped asking me. At first, I was worried he wanted to go elsewhere, but I ended up believing him when he assured me. that didn't matter much considering the love we have. "

"It is not a philosophy of life or prejudice, says Mathew. If the circumstances had been different, if we had not encountered these difficulties after the birth of our daughter, perhaps today we would have a more sexual relationship. I have not made a cross on this aspect. Of our relationship, but today it is. Also, curiously, I have the feeling that we have developed a different sensuality, which is expressed, for example, in the way we enjoy a good wine together or a meal in our favourite restaurant. What counts above all is the desire to be together, and this desire is always intense ".

Sex is a matter of impulses, but they are satisfied in various ways. The pleasures of the mouth - tasting a good wine, sharing an excellent dinner - satisfy the oral urge. Visiting an exhibition, watching a film, travelling, discovering new landscapes meet the needs of the sexual drive - the drive of the gaze. It should not be thought that these activities are only pale and weak substitutes for genital sexuality, which would be the real voice of pleasure. It is the sexual drive which, sublimated, i.e. deviated from its primary purpose, inspires artists and makes them creative.

Open to sensuality and feel better the touch, the love. We confuse sensuality and sexual pleasure, "sensoriality" and animalism. However, there are ways to reconnect to the world. This reconciliation is essential: it is our joie de vivre!

We have to distinguish between sensuality and sexuality. I see couples who do not make love in the academic sense of the term, but who continue to kiss, to touch, to cuddle: many proofs of love. By definition, I only receive couples who want to get out of this abstinence in my office. However, I am often amazed at the time they have been able to spend without suffering during their marriages.

Each massage has its specificity. Some bring only pleasure to the body; others help you relax, some even relieve various ailments or pathologies. So, you understand, we do not use massage to feel good, but also to heal. Furthermore, the types of massage we will introduce are among the most successful!

Things you need for your first erotic massage

To perform an erotic massage, you need to know how to choose the right equipment. A bed or a massage table is, for example, far from ideal to highlight sensuality in all its forms. Indeed, this piece of furniture is not suitable because it is too tall for a real sensual massage between two completely naked bodies. The idea is to practice the erotic massage on a mattress that will be installed directly on the floor, for optimal comfort, including throws, blankets, bath towels, pillows, a bed. You will have chosen flexible clothes that will allow you to move freely, fluidly and efficiently in your movements.

Accessories for an erotic massage

It is better to choose massage oil for two. If you chose coconut oil, for example, it would be a shame to learn at first that your partner has a deep dislike for its oily texture. For an erotic massage, you would prefer a dry oil that the skin absorbs quickly. Argan oil is a good base. Its light scent and its multiple virtues make it ideal for this type of massage. You can add, according to your preferences, an essential oil: jasmine subtly aphrodisiac, rose or more masculine scents such as patchouli, cedarwood and ylang-ylang. Make sure these essential oils are suitable for massages. Sandalwood oil and sweet almond oil give an ideal blend for a foot massage.

Californian massage to relax and fight various tensions

The Californian massage works by relaxing the patient, soothing his pain and awakening his body-mind awareness. It directly attacks the tensions felt by the body and mind of the person being massaged. These tensions are dissolved, thanks to the gentle and fluid movements performed by the masseur or masseur. These movements consist of brushing: the masseur touches the skin and then specifies its actions so that the tensions are relieved. This precision will also lead to awakening the memory of the person being massaged so that it determines the origin of his or her stress, which facilitates Californian massage therapy. Note that the latter is used to treat chronic ailments, muscle, joint pain and many others. The Californian massage is classified as one of the most relaxing massages, suitable for people who continuously stress or feel various tensions in their body. But be careful, there are mistakes you shouldn't make in others to get a great relaxing massage.

Chapter 10

A set of tantric sex exercises for beginners:

1. Build a special space

Move consciously from the realm of nature and enter the world of the Divine, the universe of pleasure. Turn off devices, light candles or incense, and pick up unique treatments like chocolate or berries. Purify yourself by taking a shower and dressing in beautiful things; clean up your space and put away the laundry. It is also best to forget and turn on the drugs to be fully present.

Set expectations for this intimacy session, such as "my goal is to show you how much I love you with my body" or "I am curious to receive you deeply".

1. Test eye contact/soul observation

There is nothing to hide in your partner's powerful gaze, and you practice fully disclosing yourself to the other person with all that you feel and are. You see them entirely while allowing yourself to be seen at the same time.

Sit straight on your partner's cushion or seat. You can look at your left eye and look at both eyes gently, and you can hold your hands if you wish. Let your eyes shine for love in your heart. Speaking with your wife, you see the divine spark in their eyes, marvelling at the pure life force that animates them, experience together with the sacredness of this specific moment.

Look for two minutes. Two minutes. Remember what emotions or feelings you are forced to look away; this is not a race, so you can always close your eyes for a couple of seconds and reopen them.

1. Hands-on the circuit of the heart

This can often flow well after looking at the eye. Place your hands on your heart and breathe into your heart as you sit facing each other with a gentle look. When you feel the love, your partner has in your heart, reach out and place your right hand on your partner's heart (with consent) and he can put his right hand on your heart. Each person's left hand then covers their side with their face. Pair the breath, constant, deep, nourishing. In the inhalation, you receive inspiration and love into your own body, and in the outpouring send this love down into your right arm and the heart of your friend, thus causing a chain of passion and energy to flow around you. Do this for about ten breaths.

1. Practice the yab-yum position

The classic tantric sexual disposition reflects the union of Shiva and Shakti, the two divine forces of male and female. But remember that these are just energies, and the gender of the participants doesn't matter. It is essential to practice moving from one position to another for the bonds between cis men and cis women as well.

• The base partner (Siva, energetically efficient or physically penetrating) is seated cross-legged in a "catch" position on a pillow. In contrast, the other partner (Shakti representing, who is energy efficient or physically sensitive) can rest the legs on the partner's legs with the button the bed or on a pillow or sit entirely on the partner's lap. The hands of the base partner should be around the waist of the other partner, whose legs go around the back of the base partner. Heads can be cheeky, or you can touch front to front. This position aligns the chakras of the partners and encourages the sexual energy to move along the spine. • Once aligned, take a couple of slow, deep breaths together and synchronize your breath. Then start moving in slow undulations, arching, circling, looking for an exquisite flow and rhythm that stimulates your sexual energy. The base partner "gives" the partner above who "receives" the power in his body.

• Connect to your breath to increase sexual pleasure and energy throughout the body, filling every cell with this life force. You can try to stay with smaller subtle movements or get as intense as you want, but use your breath to pull your orgasmic energy from the pelvis to the spine and third eye (the point between the eyebrows) or the crown (top) and the over there.

• This position can be performed entirely clothed, naked or in any form of penetration. You can even learn how to have full-body power orgasms, without penetration, by staying wholly clothed, but this may take a little more training!

The keys of Tantra

When we talk to people about Tantra, some are surprised. They look at us and say, "Sex for three hours? It's not possible!" The goal of Tantra is not to have a sex marathon, although this can be achieved. The goal is to forget the barriers that create a "limit" to Sex. Time is one of these barriers, where we may always be thinking about the time it should take to have Sex. How long or short should it be? Another barrier is orgasm itself, as people trying to get it to fixate on it, ignoring the other person and the act of Sex itself.

Tantra takes all the conventional concepts and focal points we have about Sex and replaces them with ideas that bring out the best this physical act can offer.

Experience

Tantra is about activating the sexual energy that we possess. In this way, we take control of our physical and emotional forces to open up a whole new dimension of Sex.

How does this change happen? One of the main goals of Tantra is to create a higher level of intimacy with your partner. The sexual aspect occurs because you share an emotional connection with your partner, and this connection is the strength you can use to make Sex something extraordinary. This force is capable of communicating many things, such as love, trust, admiration and even respect. Through the sexual act, you can convey a range of emotions.

But what about physical strength? Where does this come from? When you have emotionless Sex, then it becomes just an act of satisfying your desires and impulses. With Tantra, Sex becomes something extraordinary. Become a physical force.

You now have the emotional strength and physical strength working in total harmony, just like yin and yang. Tantra allows you to experience pleasure, love and a more peaceful state of mind.

Intimacy

Through tantric sexual experiences, you can create a more profound and more authentic connection with your partner. Develop a level of intimacy that fosters trust, understanding and love.

Sweetness

There is a sense of tenderness in Tantra that speaks volumes about the sexual act that you and your partner are engaged in. This kindness communicates respect, desire and admiration. It allows you and your partner to appreciate you to the fullest.

Slow

Sex is not rushed. Tantra reduces the speed of foreplay and intercourse. You become aware of the act and recognize every move you are making.

You are genuinely grasping the sensations, be they emotional or physical. At the same time, you gain new-found admiration and respect for your body, as well as that of your partner.

Presence

Tantra wants you to experience the joys of sex. What happened yesterday does not concern you now. What might happen in the future is best left to reflect at another time? All that matters in the present is what you and your partner are indulging in.

Sensuality

Allowing yourself and your partner to feel sensual before becoming sexual will enable you to communicate sensations between mind, body and soul. At the same time, you can enjoy a prolonged sexual experience and delay ejaculation as much as possible. All the techniques that Tantra mentions on meditation, exercises, touch and foreplay are there to help you enter a state known as "sexual meditation". In other words, when you have sex, it feels like a beautiful, meditative experience. Absorb every sensation and sensation, and this helps you enjoy sex for longer.

Ready and stable before you go

Tantra takes a holistic approach to sex. As you probably already know, Tantra is not about results, but about the journey to get there. Eventually, you may forget what you intended to achieve in the first place - such as the transformative nature of Tantra. Your environment also plays a vital role in determining your mindset, improving your ability to relax and prepare, and keep breathing and tension constant. Once you've set the mood, you're ready for the journey.

Here are some tips for enhancing tantric sex.

Temperature

Make sure your room or space has a comfortable temperature. If the room is too hot, turn on the air conditioner and set the temperature to the 70's range, which ensures that the place is cool, but not cold. For cold temperatures, turn on the heat at least an hour before you start having sex.

Lighting

You can choose to set the mood with candles or coloured light bulbs. Candles work well for adding a touch of romance, while coloured light bulbs make the space sensual and erotic. What you choose depends on the type of atmosphere you would like to create.

Perfume

You can also fill the space with a beautiful scent. You can use essential oils, scented candles, flowers, or incense sticks. It is advisable to avoid deodorants and sprays. Sticking to something a little more natural creates the right mood. Make sure you choose a scent that you and your partner both enjoy. You or your partner may be allergic to certain fragrances, so try different scents so you can find out if either of you has allergies that you both should be aware of.

Softness

Make sure the surface you choose for sex is soft. Even if you decide to pick up the floor, try to make it more comfortable by placing a soft blanket, pillows or cushions. If you are on the bed, decorate it further with pillows.

Vibrations

Enhance the sexual and romantic atmosphere by playing soft music. You may even want to dance to the music before having sex.

For your listening pleasure, we present you a tracklist to spice up your sex.

- Wicked Game by Chris Isaak
- Need You Tonight by INXS

- I'm on Fire by Bruce Springsteen

- Lay Lady Lay by Bob Dylan

- Fade Into You by Mazzy Star

- Prince's sexy MF

- Do Right Woman, Do Right Man by Arethra Franklin

- Love to Love You Baby by Donna Summer

- The Sweetest Taboo by Sade

- Usher's Climax

- I want your George Michael sex

- Feel Like Makin 'Love by Roberta Flack

- Slow Motion of Juvenile

- Pyramids of Frank Ocean

Feel free to add your favourite songs to the list or replace the file above with your collection. The idea is to create an atmosphere that you find erotic.

Before we get to the fun part

People often wonder if there is a ritual to be performed before starting tantric sex. There isn't: Tantra isn't so rigorous as to provide a specifically prescribed method for interacting with your partner. However, we have some tips to allow your sexual energy to flow freely through your body, create sexual tension, and communicate your lust to your partner. It is a good idea to practice these before your first tantric sexual experience, to ensure that you and your partner are on the same page and ready to move forward as you begin this journey together.

Eye of the beholder

Look into each other's eyes for as long as possible without blinking and try to communicate what you feel. Do you suddenly feel uncomfortable? Don't hide those feelings. Take them out. Many couples have ended up laughing uncontrollably. This is fine too. You are allowing all the emotions to come out of you. Enjoy the moment and let it continue for as long as you want. Tantra means slowing down and appreciating every moment you spend together, so don't rush to the next step - take your time and look at your partner for who they are. And make sure you allow your gaze to reflect your most profound self as well.

When you look into each other's eyes, you are letting each other know that you would like to have an exciting, enjoyable and pleasant sexual experience, but you are in no rush. For now, you are both happy to admire each other. You hold each other on a pedestal, and this is what you have to convey through your eyes. Breath of the Wild

Try to synchronize your breathing. You can do this by encouraging your partner to relax. Allow him or her to bring inspiration to a calm state. Once their breathing is regular, you can match it with yours. There is no need to rush through the process. In many cases, people may feel nervous, as what they are about to experience is new to them. There is a sense of anticipation and excitement. When you and your partner are amid all that arousal, be sure to maintain eye contact. Let each other know how much fun you are enjoying and how much you want each other. Once you've exhausted everything you would like to communicate with each other, focus on calming and synchronizing your breathing.

Touch of pleasure

Don't hesitate to tell your partner what you like. When they touch you in a certain way, or get playful with you, be open to them about whatever you'd like them to do. If specific actions have given you waves of pleasure, let your partner know they should continue and let them do the same to you. Find out what makes your partner wild. Sometimes, you don't even have to use words to say it. You can let your partner know what you like or want most by doing something to show them your feelings of pleasure. Likewise, communicate to your partner that they can feel free to use their body language to guide your touches to turn them on.

The mind of the Lover

If you have intentions specific to your sexual experience, don't be afraid to set them. You won't lower the intensity of sex in any way - in fact, determining an intention can help you get closer to your partner. However, don't stick to a particular act. For example, as we have repeated throughout the book, your goal shouldn't be to orgasm. Instead, allow your intention to swallow the whole experience. You may say that you would like to have better sex, which has a much more significant result for you and your partner - and may or may not include orgasm, in particular. You may also have emotional intentions, such as building love between you and your partner, building trust, or adding more happiness to your relationship.

When you're ready, let's take a look at Tantric Sex Positions.

Chapter 11: Tantric positions and practices

We are here to show how new joining bodies can be. Before we start exploring locations, however, it's important to note a few things:

Don't rush through the sites. Even when penetration is involved, take it slow. Feel the energy flowing through your body and enjoy the waves of pleasure. Remember that Tantra is not a wish list, in which the goal is to complete all tasks before a set deadline. Tantra does not focus on the concept of time, and it focuses on the sexual experience itself. You will have plenty of opportunities to try out all the positions, and all that Tantra has to offer, so there is no need to feel like you need to do it all at once. Focus on the feelings that accompany each experience instead of thinking ahead of what will come next.

Enjoy the freedom to switch from one location to another. This keeps things arousing and adds some surprises to the sexual experience. Also, you can change your position if you or your partner start to feel uncomfortable in a particular area. When you are tuned into the act of making love, you will instinctively know if you want to change your position. Until then, continue in the area you are currently enjoying. Your mind should focus on the act of understanding your partner. When you change your position, you create a new way of communication. Each one is like having a different conversation, exploring new ideas and thoughts.

Be aware of your partner. Look at their body. Make proper eye contact. Use sensual words during sex if you wish. But awareness also means that you should remove any distractions from your mind before having sex. This allows you to focus on your partner with all your attention. Use her arousal to feed your thirst for a different sex position. When both of you can speak like this through your sex, you have established a secure channel of communication. That said, it's also important to note the next point.

Don't feel disappointed if things don't work out correctly the first time. Your mind should be on your partner and the sexual act itself. Don't worry if you are doing something correctly or if you somehow miss it. These concerns are irrelevant. This is not an indication of your sexual prowess, abilities or character. Think of it like applying for a driver's license. You may not know how to drive the car thoroughly at first, but you know you will get there. Still, you never complained about your driving skills at first, did you? You kept improving. Sex is the same. There is no level of perfection at all. There is nothing to be "good" at. There are simple things you would like to develop with your partner and experience with him or her. Sounds good? Then let's get started.

The kiss

Start by giving your partner gentle kisses all over the body.

When you approach to kiss, don't rush. Relax your mouth and keep your kisses tender and soft. Start by kissing the top of your partner's lips before moving on to the bottom.

● You should feel as if you are massaging your partner's lips between yours. Once you press the desired boil inside you, become more passionate with your kisses.

● Pinch your partner's lips between yours. Remember, we said squeeze: don't squeeze their mouths like you're going to make pancakes out of them.

● When you are kissing, your head will likely be tilted to one side. Don't hesitate to switch sides. Gently pull your lips away from your partner's and tilt your head away, entering again for the kiss.

• Allow your partner to do the work too. This is not a demonstration of domination. Communication is a two-way street. After saying something, allow your partner to respond, also showing you his love.

• You don't even have to keep kissing your partner's lips. Gently kiss their cheek and keep kissing them until it reaches their neck. You can then bury your head in this region and gently kiss, suck and nibble your partner there. You can also gently kiss and lick your partner's ear, increasing the sexual tension between you.

• While kissing, let your hands communicate too. Run them through your partner's hair, put them on their cheek, hold their hands in yours or even cover their face.

• You don't have to be in constant contact with your partner. Let your lips part. Bring them closer to your partner's lips and exhale. Open your eyes and look deeply into your partner's. Let them know you want more.

The touch

Touch your partner and allow him or her to touch you. This will enable you to feel each other's bodies and explore them, which, if your sex life has been missing, maybe that's something you haven't done in a while. Let that connection rebuild as you communicate using only your hands. Touching each other also allows you to move slowly into a sexual position of your choice.

As always, relax. If you want to go from touching to kissing, do so. There is no urgency to jump straight into a sex position. Slow down and appreciate what it feels like to connect with your partner through the sensation of touch, showing them the intensity of your desire and passion. You could also give him a massage and work the muscles with your hands to help them relax and prepare for lovemaking.

Chapter 12

TANTRIC MASSAGE TECHNIQUES

Back rubbing is perhaps the ideal approach to relieve excess tension in the body, improve the blood flow, spread recovery energies throughout the body and thanks to the tantric back massage to sexually ignite the fire inner and the desire of your treasure! Massages can be a fantastic method of helping couples or partners with benefits demonstrate that extra closeness required for each other.

We commonly starve for contact and back massage is a quaint and straightforward approach to meeting this need.

Sounds great, doesn't it?

So how to start?

All in all, gaining overly exceptional approval or significantly appropriate preparation for performing tantric back massages is generally not critical, even though what is essential is the expectation and desire to satisfy the recipient, for example, yours sincerely—accomplice through the multifaceted limits of your body (mostly hands).

Before starting with the systems, give up what tantric back rub is, how it counteracts the different types of back rub and some of the key benefits related to it. The tantric back massage as we probably know today was created from a wide range of sources, predominantly the blend of tantric thinking with the impacts of convincing Western scholars.

The characterizing highlights of the tantric back massage are:

• Tantric back rubbing revolves around the potential and use of your sexual vitality to benefit you rather than limit you.

• The expulsion of blocks in a wide range of measurements of your cognition, body, psyche and soul

• The enhancement or elevation of sexual and orgasmic encounters

• The clothes are not worn during the back rub, so the private parts are exposed most of the time.

• Spiritual arousal is the valid and extreme goal of tantra and thus of the tantric back massage

Benefits of Tantric Massage

Like a wide range of back massages, the tantric way has numerous inherent benefits as well as a few extras that make tantra somewhat progressively extraordinary.

 Currently, part of the many inherent benefits of back massage are:

• Greater prosperity

• Improved temperament

• Improved well-being and stamina

• Relief from agony, nervousness and stress

Some selective benefits that are particularly identified with tantric back rubbing are:

• Improved moxie and sex drive

• More exceptional sexual encounters

• Higher otherworldly awareness (if done effectively)

Here are some tips and systems laid out to help you get started with a tantric back massage.

PREPARATION FOR MASSAGE

For some who have never met it before, the possibility of a tantric back massage is routinely fascinating, if not downright frightening. Some would dare to see it as unthinkable, which is a severe and significant thing.
Then again, people who are aware of it think it is a unique, energizing and indispensable practice that can make reflections for the prosperity of one and those who are accomplices. Since many people don't understand what tantric back massage is and how it works, they don't see it as an alternative to solidify in their lives.

For the ideal tantric rubbing session, accomplices should take turns kneading each other. As previously mentioned, this type of back massage requires the recipient to be open and responsive, and indulging in the experience is commonly the ideal approach.

In case you have little self-confidence or are simply too self-conscious, the tantric back massage can show you how to recognize, love and enjoy yourself more. Likewise, it can help increase your accomplice's certainty as you appreciate closeness to that person and help them feel known and loved for who they are.

To get started, here are some things you should do before starting the procedure:

- Prepare your space

Prepare the room or any area you need to use, be it a living room or a private place, with many delicate pads and open to bedding. Put some lit and on the off chance that you want marginally scented candles, scattered around the room - away from combustible things. Keep your lighting entirely off or at the dimmest customizable level.

Pour drinking water or wine into a reflective glass on hand with the aim that it will be useful and enjoyable for you. You may also need to put in a few light bites to maintain vitality or to support each other. If you need the room to smell delicious, you may need to use a base oil diffuser with a fresh, soothing aroma.

-Be ready physically, mentally and spiritually

Before you begin, allow yourself to have an open heart and a receptive perspective. If something, in particular, is causing you discomfort, it is generally best to ignore them, but equally, it can be great to work on some of the things that lead to this inclination. The most widely recognized discomfort one encounters regularly is due to weakness and unfavourable reluctance towards specific highlights in one's body. During practice, it is essential to maintain a lively mood and show enthusiasm for discovering new types of a beautiful collaboration.

Before the session begins, it may be necessary to scrub or shower, improving, but maintaining a strategic distance from the sexual association during that time. Stand up close and personal and stretch anyway, you better give up on any effort.

Wear nice clothes. Make sure your clothes, shorts, underwear and shirt are free enough for a simple ejection. In any case, wearing them without wearing anything would also be an incredible choice. Be that as it may, since tantra is about a moderate gathering of sexual vitality, it's generally a smart thought to start with your clothes.

-Begin the process by slowly building the sexual energy

After doing some stretching and washing the dishes, throw yourself in front of each other and be kind. You should sit with your legs bent or put your legs on top of each other all together because of the vitality of the erogenous zones close to each other.

Look at each other for at least five minutes: it is said that the eyes are the windows of the spirit, and this applies to this circumstance. You may think it's embarrassing from the start, however, keep looking into your eyes for as long as possible. The moment you feel that all pressures wither without end, a genuine association has been built. This is the goal. This is the real feeling of association you need to discover in Tantric sex. Try to make propensity to keep your eye-to-eye connection throughout the practice.

START OF THE TANTRIC MASSAGE

Here are several basic massage strategies that are pleasing to the student that you can perform directly.

- Start with your backside

About two tablespoons of oil should be enough to start. Smear the oil on your hands first and then start rubbing your hands to warm the palm. At that point, place your hands on your sweetie's lower back and allow your hands to crawl along the end of your affection through the neck, anywhere on the shoulders and back, anywhere in the back area.

- The Hand Slide

Since you have the oil on your better half's back, start running your fingers along the spine, kneading up to the lower back and over the rump. Go up to the neck, at that point on the shoulders, and then the arms and fingertips. Repeat in each case several times. As you stage it, speak with your affection and ask if he feels like it's criticism. Your significant other is of the non-talking type; you don't need to coerce the person in question. Remember that it is related to giving your accomplice a feeling of prosperity and relaxation.

- "Force Ups"

For a change, try turning hand after hand as you approach and rub the side of your sweetie's body. Start by placing both hands on your hips and then gently pull them down to your spine.

Move your hands to the central part and take it down to the spine. At that point, place your hands on your chest and return to the spine. Find your hands just under your armpits and take them down to your spine. Make sure you do the two parts.

- Massage

On the off chance that you prepare yourself, at that point, this strategy would be easy (no pun intended.) However, in case you haven't, you can squeeze your darling's back and shoulders between your thumb and several fingers in a crooked motion using one hand and then the other. Then, coast your hands on another part of the back and repeat the same procedure until your accomplice has been well worked, starting from the neck to the end. The fleshy parts of the body, for example, the hindquarters could bear more weight, along these lines, don't stress yourself out to squeeze it a little harder and marginally spread your cheeks as you exercise. This will make your accomplice excited.

- Goose stroke

Before moving onto your thighs, stroke your accomplice's neck, arms, shoulders, back and back using your fingertips in a very light stroke. Do this for about five minutes. In case your nails are long, gently scratch your accomplice's skin. You can do this in round motions, from side to side. Take into consideration your light, prickly contacts and caresses create erotic arousal for your sweetheart as they wouldn't understand which part of their body you are about to contact immediately.

- Foot Care

Maybe you will need more oil on this one. Add more oil to your hand, scrub your hands, and put more oil on your accomplice's body. At the moment, the hand glide technique on the thigh begins just as the calf moves gradually. Begin to execute the manipulator once more, followed by a lighter one. Do one leg at once. Significantly, the feet are an incredibly erogenous zone, so you need to give them some deep regard! Put more oil on each foot, rubbing it all over the lower leg, at that point at the point of impact and into the toes. With your palms, slide the base of your accomplice's foot back and forth several times. Rotate your accomplice's toes clockwise and then counterclockwise and finally slide your index finger between each tip. Gently pull each tip away from your body.

- Transform your lover

At this point, your accomplice is undoubtedly satisfied with what you simply did on their backs. Now continue focusing on the front area of your accomplice. Once again, put more oil in your hand and then smear it on the button of your loved one's belly, running it continuously towards the centre of the stomach and all the areolas, at that point to the button of the intestine of your accomplice. Do it again and again because your accomplice will appreciate it and spread vitality over their body. In case your sweetie is a girl, try to be cautious when you are on her breasts right now. The male can tolerate more forceful blows. All in all, you can do a massage on the male's chest.

Chapter 13

DIFFERENT POSITIONS OF TANTRIC / YOGA

When you are finally ready to take it to the next level, there is essential tantric back rub positions ideal for amateurs. Depending on your level of adaptability, you can change positions according to your preferences and comfort. The most significant thing is to focus on the association and the time you spend with your accomplice and appreciate each other's closeness. Ideally, you will experience a higher bond in a calm state. Start at your agreeable level, impart your varying degrees of adaptability and quality, and most notably practice a deep face-to-face connection, feeling each one's dash and positive reflections on each other without saying a single word.

The following are some tantric postures you can try with your lover:

1. Yab Yum

This posture is useful for regulating vitality between couples. An accomplice sits serenely with his legs bent on a tangle. Then the other accomplice sits on the other's thighs and crosses the lower legs behind the accomplice. Use your stomach and lower back muscles to stay straight and aligned with each other. Make your contact and inhale seriously and gradually reliably. You can do this posture with your eyes closed or open.

In performing this posture, I would prescribe you to travel through these three stages to build a protected space and to console the vigorous passion for gradually modelling. Each "session" must last 20 minutes. Remember to set a clock, so you don't have to stress over time as you go through the process.

Phase 1: Both you and your accomplices must demonstrate Easy Pose by confronting each other with knees touching gently. Put your hands on each other's knees. Look into each other's eyes without focusing on anything in the room. Hinder your breathing example until your breaths synchronize. Quietly organize a breathing musicality that you know both of you enjoy.

Phase 2: You and your accomplice open your legs. The lady should sit as close to her accomplice as possible, folding her legs over his hand over his lower back. Place your hands on each other's middle or shoulders. Even putting your hands on the mother's heart would be a choice. As in the initial step, it is equally essential to observe your breathing example.

Phase 3: The last position of this posture is the exemplary position that appears in the photo above. The lady sits on the lap of her accomplice. Start comparing yourself with eyebrows touching and arms serene around each other. Now you should still look at each other in the eye; the eye-to-eye connection gradually transforms into an expanded physical touch as you focus on relaxation.

Notice the nature of the vitality now. How does it feel? In which part of your body do you think it? Allow him to move without reservations. Give your organs a chance to grasp fully. Right now, the lady's feminine vitality, just like her innovative life power and kundalini, are creating together.

1. Position of the boat

In this posture, you will use your core muscles. This is a decent posture for extending and fortifying. This is also yoga which represents that if done alone and wrongly, it could give you low back agony assuming you don't have stomach quality, your lower back muscles will try to keep you in high equalization, but this risk is less when you end up with an accomplice. Also, you can regulate it by relying on your comfort and adaptability.

Phase 1: Sit on the floor facing each other with your legs forward and your knees slightly bent.

Phase 2: With your knees bent, go on until and put the soles of your feet at your accomplice's feet and get into each other's hands. Lean your back and push your feet against your accomplices.

Phase 3: Gently stretch your legs and, however, keeping your feet in contact.

Step 4: In the request to develop the association, twist the knees gradually, keeping the sole in its position, and after which move the legs independently on the two sides of. Extend your knees again with your legs out of your arms.

1. Downward dog

At the moment, if pot posture isn't your thing as you think you're not adaptable enough, this is a more straightforward posture, ideal for newbies. This is one of the best choices for many couples. You will feel great by curving your spine and simultaneously extending your abs and chest as your accomplice. Since it includes adjustment, getting into position can be a test, but it's far from challenging to achieve.

Here are how you do this:

Phase 1: Both started in the table position; facing each other. Get back to that position about 5 to 6 inches, tucking your toes under, so that the balls of your feet don't touch the floor.

Phase 2: As you exhale, lift your butt bones upward and bring your body into a slippery V shape, so that you are both in a downward-facing dog position.

Phase 3: Gradually walk upright and with your hands back until it is easy for you to walk on the sides of your lower back. Stop when you uncover your hips, and you can stay in place gently.

Step 4: Communicate as your feet move forward to make sure they don't harm and to maintain your association.

Step 5: Stay in that position for 5-7 breaths, at which point your accomplice should gradually rotate their knees, lowering their hips to the table position and after that guy's posture as you tenderly drop your feet to the ground. You can do this again by exchanging points.

This is a primary inversion that transmits length into the spine. It is equally extraordinary in enhancing correspondence and closeness.

1. Seated Twisting

This is a tantric back rub where you both need to sit with your legs bent, facing each other. The spinal curves posture is known to be a real relaxation gift when performed alone, however, when presented with your accomplice, this posture might not just improve your devilish spines and soothe your general inclination, but additionally, it can initiate the vicinity.

This is how you can reproduce this tantric massage position:

Phase 1: Sit in a comfortable position facing each other; your knees should make contact with each other.

Phase 2: Sit straight with your body slightly forward, shoulders lose and jawline pointing down.

Phase 3: Put your left ArmArm behind your back and extend your other ArmArm. Get your accomplice to do something very similar.

Step 4: Reach for your accomplice's left hand using the right side while offering your left hand to your accomplice's right hand. This position will transform your body which is your goal.

Step 5: Slowly curve your body as much as you need; however, make sure you are both pleasant. Maintain consistent correspondence throughout the process.

Step 6: Stay in this position anyway for two minutes, then switch sides.

1. Lower arm support

Lower ArmArm The support supports the shoulders, core and arms just like the back and extends the shoulders and chest. This tantric posture likewise strengthens and fortifies the body, improves proprioception and balance, and creates a high blood flow. It is an incredible posture for practising balance and bringing out the confidence in your lover.

This posture is an incredible practice to do alone, but better if finished with an accomplice; here's the way you do it.

Phase 1: Perform a side position on the floor and noticeably relax all around and have your accomplice hold your legs when they are high enough to bring your body upright.

Phase 2: when your accomplice has both legs, and you finally feel stable, urge him to place one with his hands clenched in the centre of the lower limbs. Request that your accomplice let go gradually and you should be able to remain floating in case you hold the hug of your inner thighs including the wrist.

To unload, ask your accomplice to squeeze your hips, with the ultimate goal that you can rotate from the hips as you descend.

In conclusion, the tantric massage can be an extraordinarily satisfying and satisfying knowledge; physically and rationally as well as intensely. To be sure, the otherworldly point of view is arguably the most significant. In case you are passionate about other rubbing methods and the real benefits that can be obtained from rubbing on the back, do not hesitate to examine those items as well.

Chapter 14

Sex

Scissors

This pose is unique in that you will not be using the bed, but a raised surface such as a kitchen counter or table. As this is the first of many of these positions, we hope you have a sturdy table to endure your actions!

The woman lies down, her back pressed against the surface of the platform or table. You can also try your bed. The man will have to lean forward to lean slightly, but this shouldn't cause him any discomfort. If it feels uncomfortable, the couple should use another raised platform. Whichever surface the couple chooses, the woman's pelvis should be slightly lower than the man's. He should then lift his legs and place them on the man's shoulders.

Before the man penetrates, he should put his hands under his hips. This will also give him the freedom to hold her buttocks and adjust the thrust angle.

Sexual suggestion

• Since the man can hold the woman's buttocks, he can gently squeeze them while thrusting to add some excitement and tease the woman a little!

• The woman can use her hands to stimulate herself by gently rubbing her clitoris. This not only increases his pleasure, but it also turns him on even more.

#The Couch Lean

For this position, you should use a sofa or chair, whichever you feel comfortable with or is available.

The man should be sitting on the sofa. The woman should straddle him, with her legs apart as she brings her knees to his chest. Then, carefully, the woman should lean back, making sure she feels comfortable doing this. He can also stretch his arms behind him and touch the floor if he can.

The man can then enter the woman and control the thrusts.

Sexual suggestion

● The woman can also take control of this position. He can rest his hands on the floor and, using them to maintain balance, push himself back and forth against the man.

The tugboat

This is a unique position and will require the couple to be lying on the bed or other comfortable surface.

The man should sit cross-legged, and the woman should lie on him. She should then gently lower herself onto his erection and wrap her legs around him.

When the couple is sitting face to face, they should hold each other by the elbows and, using those elbows as leverage, lean back. From this position, the couple can manage their thrusts.

If partners are feeling particularly flexible, they may even lean back to the surface of the bed. Couples shouldn't try this move unless they are confident.

#The Wall Press

A popular standing position, this one never fails to drive the couple crazy with ecstasy! It is important to note that the man may require good upper body strength. If the couple is unsure of this position, they shouldn't attempt it.

The woman should start by leaning against a wall, facing her man, and spread her legs slightly.

The man should then grab her thighs, bringing them closer to her hips, then lift the woman and lean her against the wall.

It should lean against the wall for convenience. At this point, the man can push himself into the woman.

#The Side Hold

The couple should lie sideways on the bed or any other smooth surface, facing each other.

The woman should wrap her legs around the man's legs, which allows him to penetrate deep inside her.

To achieve balance, the couple can hold on to each other, increasing the intimacy of the position.

The reverse thrust

To initiate this position, the woman should lie on her back and pull her knees up to her chest.

Once this is done, the man kneels before the woman. At this point, it looks like her buttocks are slightly raised. The man then holds the woman's feet as he penetrates her.

Sexual suggestion

• The couple can make this position even more exciting: the woman can place her feet on the man's chest, and he can hold her hips while he pushes.

#The victory pose

The woman should make herself comfortable on a table or counter. The man should be facing her, and she should start the pose by placing her hands on his shoulders. The man should then bring his arms to her lower back to prepare her for the next move.

He should then lift his right leg and place the foot or leg on his shoulder. Once his right leg is comfortably positioned, he can perform the same move with his left leg.

Sexual suggestion

• The woman can hold the man's face to increase the intensity of the position. Alternatively, she can run her hands through his hair or over his head to encourage him to take it slow. It entirely depends on the couple!

The climb

As this is another standing position to spice up the sexual experience, keep in mind that it may take some practice to get it right. If the couple is unable to perform in this position on the first try, there is no need to feel disappointed or frustrated. Instead, use the moment to share a laugh and enjoy the fact that you are making mistakes together.

The couple can stand anywhere in the room and can use the wall for extra support if needed.

If the couple is standing in the centre of the room, the man should put his arms on the woman's back as she lifts one of her legs and wraps it around her. This way, he will stand on one leg.

If the couple is leaning against a wall, the man will have his hands free to touch her face or run them through her hair.

Sexual suggestion

• If the woman can be even more flexible, she can lift her legs and rest them on the man's shoulders.

The Lean Back

To begin, the woman should lie down on the bed or a soft surface. He should then lift the lower body, supporting the upper body with the shoulders and forearms. The man should kneel in front of her, holding her thighs, and enter her. Be careful not to get out of bed!

The hops

This location is for those who would like to experience something truly adventurous. It is also important to point out that this position requires the woman to have a high degree of flexibility.

Lying on her back, she should bend her legs so that they go over her head. Eventually, he should find that his toes touch the floor above his head. The woman can lift her body to reach this position, keeping balance on her head and shoulders. He can place his arms on his hips or use them as additional support.

Once the woman is ready, the man can squat on her and penetrate her. It is this unusual position that makes sex even more sparkling.

Sexual suggestion

● The man can choose to "dip" his penis in and out, which allows him to tease the woman before pushing himself inside her.

The comfortable cowgirl

If you're not in the mood to try something that requires you to put your back on like the previous position, try this move.

When the man is sufficiently comfortable lying on a bed or other suitable surface, the woman should sit on him with her knees planted on either side. After gently lowering herself on her erection, she should use her pelvis to control movement in two ways:

● Can lean forward slightly and move back and forth. ● Or, she could sit upright and bounce up and down.

Sexual suggestion

● The woman can spread her knees and then bring them back together if she wants. This makes the position even more exciting.

The bow

This is another pose that may require some degree of flexibility. The man will sit on the bed with his legs stretched out in front of him. The woman will slowly approach him, building the sexual tension, to gently straddle his erect penis.

Once they are comfortable, it arches backwards. Women must be careful at this point so as not to put unnecessary strain on the back. If they feel discomfort while having sex in this position, do not proceed further. After all, there is no shortage of sexual situations in this book.

When the woman arches back, she should do so until she can hold her ankles. The man will then lean forward and start pushing inside her. You will be able to enjoy the sight of the woman's body erotically arching backwards, and she can experience all the thrusts of the man.

Sexual suggestion

● To add more excitement to the position, the man can lean forward and gently kiss or cup the woman's breasts, or place his hands on her back.

● If he can, he can lean forward and enjoy a passionate kiss with his partner. While leaning back, the couple can look at each other in the eye until the woman has to lean back to hold her ankles.

Freedom

This is a fun pose that allows the woman to stretch her legs while the man does the work. To begin, the woman should lie down on a soft surface with her legs apart. The man should then reach down and gently penetrate the woman, but he should not proceed with the thrust yet.

The woman should then lift her legs and place them on either side of the man. Once her legs are straight, the woman should simply let them relax. The man can support them by placing his hands under or above the knees. Once the couple is comfortable, the man can start pushing into the woman.

To make things comfortable for the woman, she can put her hands at her hips or behind her head.

The sleeping dog

Lying face down on a soft surface, the woman should lift her buttocks slightly, using her knees and hands to bring balance and comfort to the position.

The man should get down and penetrate her.

Sexual suggestion

● Man can spice things up by grabbing a woman's buttocks. Or he could bend over, reach under her, and cup her breasts. To enjoy this position longer, the man should take deep breaths and use shallow thrusts.

The lifting

This position is similar to the previous one, but with a small modification. The woman should get on her hands and knees on the bed, gently resting her head on a pillow or soft surface. His arms should be placed in a comfortable position. In this way, she will lean forward with her buttocks raised. Man can, therefore, use this opportunity to penetrate it.

Sexual suggestion

● The woman can easily stimulate her clitoris while the man penetrates her.

The Soft Wrap

The woman should lie on the bed on one side and lift the leg of the team that is not touching the bed. For example, if the woman is lying on her left hand, she should raise her right leg.

The man can then enter the woman from behind, and once he does, the woman should wrap her raised leg around the man's side. The couple should maintain eye contact as the man pushes himself into the woman.

Sexual suggestion

● The man can use his hands to stimulate the woman's clitoris, giving her an extra dose of pleasure. If the man positions himself correctly, he could encourage her clitoris with one hand and gently caress her breasts with the other.

The final round

For this position, the man will sit on the edge of the bed or, if the couple is feeling adventurous, on the stairs or the side of the bathtub. A fair warning to those who choose to use the tub for this position: be careful and make sure you have a right balance. Also, check that the edge of the container is dry so that it offers a firmer grip for the man's buttocks.

Once the man is seated, the woman should lower on his erection. But here's the twist: she should sit across from him. This way, she becomes free to control the action.

Sexual suggestion

● The woman can arch her back and lean on the man. You can choose to run your hand through his hair or put it on the back of his neck.

● The man can create intensity by placing one of his hands on the woman's chest and using the other left to caress her thighs. He can wet her neck with soft kisses or suck it gently. To send waves of pleasure through her, he can also nibble on the woman's ear.

The informal seating

This position almost makes it seem as if the couple is simply sitting on the bed to relax. Therefore, if you prefer something less intense, but still different, this position is ideal.

The man will sit down first, with one of his legs on the bed and the other dangling. He can lean back and balance on his arms if that makes him more comfortable. The woman will then lower onto his penis, but will face the other way. He can adjust his position to feel comfortable. This gives everyone the ability to change the speed of the action.

Sexual suggestion

● With their hands-free, the couple can explore each other's body. For example, the man can lean forward and gently massage the woman's clitoris while she can play with her scrotum. We have a feeling that both of you will ask for more!

The push-up

The pair will require good upper body strength for this position. With the woman kneeling on the floor on all fours, the man should stand behind her. He will then grab her legs and lift her buttocks to her waist, allowing her to balance on her hands as if she were about to do a push-up. He can then start pushing inside her, controlling the pace and intensity.

Sexual suggestion

• Before trying this, check that both of you will feel comfortable having sex in this position. To do this, the woman should get on all fours, and the man should try to lift her slightly. He should see if he feels an effort and the woman should make sure that she does not feel any discomfort, neither in the arms nor in the upper body. Only when they are ready should they proceed further.

• If the couple has decided to feel comfortable experiencing this sexual position, the man can further stimulate the woman by massaging her clitoris as he pushes them inside. The intensity will take your breath away!

The pose

The woman should lie on her side near the edge of the bed as if posing for a painting. Her back should be facing the man, and she should balance her upper body on her arm. She should then press her thighs together as the man lowers himself on her from behind, entering her softly and slowly. When she starts pushing, the woman should keep her legs slightly crossed.

Sexual suggestion

• With this position, the man has the freedom to explore the woman's body. He can shower her with sensual touches and kisses or run your fingers along her hips and arms. He can even lift one of his legs to increase the intensity by a few notches.

#The mould

The couple sits on the bed, facing each other. If desired, the couple can increase the sexual tension before entering the position by holding each other's gaze like this for a while. Then they will lean back on their hands and slowly move their hips towards each other until penetration. Man or woman can control the speed of making love.

Sexual suggestions

● If the couple is feeling adventurous, they can switch from The Mold to a cowgirl position. Start by approaching each other, as if they are about to hug. Hence, the man can slowly lean back until he is lying on his back. The woman can proceed to check the speed and intensity of the movement. She can put her hands on the man's chest while he can gently massage her breasts. This change of position improves sexual experience.

caster

In this position, the man lies on his back, keeping his legs slightly apart and his arms extended beside him. Once ready, the woman lowers herself face down on the man, stretching her body to fit the man's position. Then gently slide down his body and onto his erection, using his arms to move up and down.

Sexual suggestions

● The man can cup the woman's face with his hands as they look deeply into her eyes. Couples can also indulge in soft or passionate kisses, making the moment incredibly romantic and exciting.

● If you have massage oils, apply them to each other's body. You can start with a little massage to relax your partner and set the mood. The couple should make sure that the massage oil does not cover the man's penis, as it will penetrate the woman. Otherwise, you are free to explore!

Facedown

In this position, the woman lies face down on the bed, with her upper body extending beyond the surface of the bed. This way, he'll lean face down towards the floor, using his hands to balance himself.

The man will do all the work as he approaches the woman from behind and thrusts inside her. She can place her hands on her hips to keep her balance, but if the woman feels too much pressure, she can lean forward with her palms planted on the surface of the bed as if she were going to do push-ups.

Sexual suggestion

• When we say that man does all the work, we mean that man does all the job. This implies that he can lean forward and plant sensual kisses on the woman's back, nibble her ear gently, or even use one of his arms to grab the woman's buttocks while using the other to balance himself.

• Keep in mind that when the man is leaning forward, he may have to use the edge of the bed for support. Alternatively, he can place his arms on the floor next to the woman, but he should only do so if he knows he is not adding pressure to the woman's body or causing both of them to position themselves in an awkward angle. After all, the couple can get out of bed, and while it may sound funny, we're more concerned about the couple getting hurt.

#The closure

The man should first sit on the bed with his legs stretched out in front of him. The woman should get down on her knees and slowly crawl towards him, creating a state of increased sexual tension. Then she straddles him, gently lowering herself on his erection.

The man takes over from here, placing his hands on her back and allowing her to lean back, making sure to use her hands for support. Careful to avoid tugging on his muscles while leaning back, she can slowly take him to a final position, at which point the man will hold his position firmly. The woman is free to raise her hands above her head and let the man do the work, keeping her knees on either side of the man to lock him in sexual surrender. When the man starts pushing himself into the woman, he can lean forward and use his mouth to stimulate her breasts.

The side step

This position offers the couple an excellent opportunity to maintain eye contact. To enter this pose, the woman will need to lie on her side. She can support the weight of her upper body with her hands, or she can choose to place her hands under her head, whichever is more comfortable for her.

She will then lift one of her legs and rest it on her lover's shoulder. The other leg is still on the bed or floor she is lying on.

The man can then penetrate the woman, allowing himself to use soft and gentle thrusts in the beginning. Another variation of this position is where the man lies behind the woman. For this reason, his legs cannot be placed on his shoulder; however, the man can use his hands to support the woman's raised legs. For some couples, it may take a few moments to find a comfortable seat before the man can penetrate.

The spread

This position gives the man strength and allows him to control the speed and depth of movements. The woman simply has to let the man do the work and enjoy the fruits of his labour.

To begin, the woman will lie on her side, tilting her body slightly so that her breasts are resting on the bed or surface. He can let his feet fall off the couch or, if the couple is lying on the floor, take them to rest on the floor.

The man will then position himself behind the woman and enter her. He can also lift her legs slightly and hold them to give him more comfortable as he penetrates the woman. In this way, the man can start softly and increase the intensity of the thrusts as the couple progresses more and more into a passionate sexual act.

The Sit Down

For this position, the woman gains control. The man can relax and feel the pleasure of moving through his body as his partner does the work.

The man should lie on his back on the bed or a soft surface with his hands resting above his head.

The woman should stand on top of the man and comfortably extend her legs until his feet are on either side of his shoulders. He can place his hands on either side or behind her while leaning back. She should then position herself so that the man's penis penetrates her.

Using the floor as a lever, the woman should begin rotating her hips in a figure-of-eight motion. She can start slowly to see if the man is comfortable, making sure his rocking movements are gentle. When the pleasure increases and the couple would like to take it a step further, the woman can gently move her hips up and down to focus on penetration. He can adjust the speed and intensity of the thrusts according to the situation.

The Yab Yum

One of the most popular positions for Tantric sex is the Yab Yum. The place itself is relatively easy to achieve and also encourages the couple to orgasm at the same time. The couple can stimulate all the right areas and enjoy the higher sexual intensity. The position also leaves the man's hands-free to explore the woman's body. He can touch his lover's body as he pleases, discovering sensitive spots, or only making her happy by showering her with physical attention. While the couple will face each other, they can even add passionate kisses to their lovemaking experience.

The man should sit cross-legged on the bed or a soft surface, keeping his back straight. The woman then straddles him as she wraps her legs around him. When the couple is comfortable, the woman can gently lower herself onto the man's penis. Here's where this position improves.

Typically, the woman takes charge of the speed and intensity of the thrusts. But if she likes it, she can give the man control. When this happens, the man can open his legs and stretch them in front of him. He can then lean back and balance his upper body on his hands, which allows him to push up. The woman will have to relax her legs so that they do not surround the man. She can still hold it, with her legs touching the man's hips, or she can stretch her legs, depending on what she finds comfortable with.

The man may also change his position if he feels that sitting cross-legged might be slightly uncomfortable.

The race

For this position, the man will lie on his back. The woman will look away from him, straddling him as she places her hands on his hips. If the man feels that the pressure on his hips is too intense, then he can put his hands close to his bones. Start with a little tease. It can slide down from the man, each time approaching the penis but not allowing penetration. The woman can even touch the man's penis with her vaginal opening, allowing the couple to engage in a little foreplay to increase sexual tension before penetration. When ready, the woman can slide towards the man's penis.

She can lean back, letting her hands rest on the man's hips and her back resting on his chest.

Sexual suggestion

● The man can cover the woman's breasts with his hands and even touch the woman's clitoris, increasing the sexual intensity of the position.

• The woman may perform some slow thrusts while leaning back against the man's chest; then she will sit down to pick up the pace. Each time he leans back, slows down to increase the tension. She can also take advantage of the position and gently massage the man's testicles. It will drive him crazy, in the right way, of course.

Sexual suggestion

• The man can tease the woman by gently exhaling on her breasts before using his tongue to explore them. He can run his tongue around her areolas or suck her breasts to send her into another realm of pleasure.

The chance encounter

This position allows the woman to lean back and enjoy it while the man gets to work. The man should lie down on the bed, his head resting on a pillow.
The woman will lower on his erection. He then leans back on his hands, placing one of his legs on the man's chest. The man should then push himself up into the woman, using his free hands to explore her body. Sexual suggestion

• The man can hold the woman's legs as a lever to control the speed and intensity of the thrusts, but the woman can take control of them at any time. He simply has to place one of his hands on the man's chest to indicate that he should calm down. Then, after returning his hand to the support position, he can move up and down his erection. By arching the back, it can create a feeling of intense sexual intensity.

• The man can reach out and hold the woman's breasts or around her waist.

The missionary

This excellent position is elegant and straightforward, which couples can get into quickly. In this position, the woman should lie down on the bed or a soft surface, separating her legs to allow the man to enter. He can start by gently placing his hands under the woman's knees, teasing her with anticipation, then slowly approach the woman until penetration, making sure he penetrates her gently.

Sexual suggestion

• The man can create tension by slowly kissing the woman's inner thigh, starting near her knees and moving towards her vaginal opening. Then, he can switch to the other leg, repeating the process there.

#

The missionary switch

In this form of a missionary, the roles are reversed, with the woman over the man. To begin, he should lie on his back with his legs open. She moves closer to him, slowly reaching his erection and leaning forward until his face is close to hers. Then slide up and down, controlling the rhythm of making love.

Sexual suggestions

Couples can add some romance by kissing now and then, and the man can run his hands through the woman's hair.

The corner of love

One of the reasons this position is so perfect is that the angle at which the woman lies down allows the man to hit the G-spot.

Reclining on her back, she should apply weight to her upper body, particularly her shoulders, and lift her buttocks, balancing her lower body using her feet. She should then invite the man by opening her legs wide, giving him a good view of her vagina.

The man then kneels between her legs and holds them in support as he penetrates her, controlling the intensity of the thrusts.

Sexual suggestions

● This is an incredible opportunity for the man to stimulate the woman's clitoris with his tongue. Next, you will find a section dedicated to helping men discover the best way to do this.

● The man should make sure to hold her legs firmly and allow the woman to balance on his hands, as it relieves some of the pressure on her.

#The Hopper

For this position, the man should have a strong core and be somewhat flexible, as he will bend his body quite athletically.

Lying on the bed, he will raise his bent legs to his chest, keeping them slightly apart and using his hands to hold the legs in place. The woman should then look away from him and lower himself on his erection. She can bounce up and down to control love and eventually allow him to hit her G-spot.

The front hopper

This position is a variation of the previous one, with the difference that the woman will face the man. Again, he controls the flow of love, but he can make it romantic by holding her hands. If she can lean forward enough, the man can take her face in his hands, and she can put her hands on her chest.

Lower placement

The man should sit right on the edge of the bed while the woman is astride him, facing the opposite direction. Once she feels comfortable, she can slowly bend down until her hands touch the floor, then push her legs back behind her. Then use your hands for leverage as you lift your hips up and down.

Making love can be made even more intense with the man touching her back. He can also place his palms on the woman's sides, allowing her to balance. The Flipper

This is a rather playful position in which the woman can indulge in some extra fun. Facedown on the bed or a soft surface, he should lift his hips with his hands under his shoulders to maintain balance and knees holding the angle of the body.

The man will then penetrate her from behind and, while doing so, the woman will be able to bend her legs to touch his back, caress him and show him how flexible he is. If the woman is unable to reach the man's end, she can lean back slightly to allow her feet to meet his skin if she so chooses.

He can also increase sexual tension at first by slowly approaching her and kissing her legs first, even starting with her feet if she wants. He can move them down her legs, thighs and finally plant soft kisses on her buttocks.

#The wide-angle

This position is designed for those who are flexible and have a strong core. The woman should lie down on the bed and lift her legs until she can place them on either side of her head.

The man will then enter the woman using the classic missionary position.

He can push the woman so that her crotch makes contact with her clitoris.

Alternatively, he can push himself from a low angle so he can hit his G-spot.

The spoon

The main ingredient of this position is romance. It allows couples to pamper themselves while enjoying their sexual experience.

The woman should lie on her side on the bed. The man will then lie down behind the woman, bringing his arms around her waist. From that position, he will penetrate her.

The couple can make it even more romantic by holding hands during intercourse or more erotic by having the man massage the clitoris.

#The Bendover

This allows the couple to enjoy sex without having to find a surface to lie on or use to sit on - perfect for a quickie if they feel like it. The woman simply needs to lean forward as much as possible, keeping her hands at her hips. The man approaches from behind and holds her hands as he penetrates her.

Control can be given to both man and woman: he can control lovemaking through the speed of his thrusts, while the woman can take command through the movement of her hips.

Properly and uses his hands for support.

Conclusion

It is not easy to explain these strong feelings even after having lived them. The tantric sex takes over and spreads mental and physical pleasures with caring and professional human physical interaction in such a sensual way.

Tantric sex is not just about touching and caressing, but also about massive conception and unique breathing methods. In unison, they create a significant impact on a person's physical, emotional and spiritual levels. This form of massage offers many health benefits, ranging from purely physical ones, such as increased immunity and stress relief, to psychological problems and healing of mental suffering. This form of massage is a great way to withhold more exceptional discernment of sexuality and develop healthier, stronger, and more intimate relationships between two lovers.

But it's not just this. The tantric sex can also be the way for an indescribable spiritual pleasure, the entrance to the Numinoso, which takes you through the limits of time and space to the sweet grip of love and harmony of the universe.

CPSIA information can be obtained
at www.ICGtesting.com
Printed in the USA
BVHW012145280521
608097BV00008B/854